MW00513205

Keto Die Cookbook 2021

Super Simple Ketogenic Recipes To Burn Fat And Lose Weight

Miranda Young

© Copyright 2021 - All rights reserved.

The content contained within this book may not be reproduced, duplicated or transmitted without direct written permission from the author or the publisher.

Under no circumstances will any blame or legal responsibility be held against the publisher, or author, for any damages, reparation, or monetary loss due to the information contained within this book. Either directly or indirectly.

Legal Notice:

This book is copyright protected. This book is only for personal use. You cannot amend, distribute, sell, use, quote or paraphrase any part, or the content within this book, without the consent of the author or publisher.

Disclaimer Notice:

Please note the information contained within this document is for educational and entertainment purposes only. All effort has been executed to present accurate, up to date, and reliable, complete information. No warranties of any kind are declared or implied. Readers acknowledge that the author is not engaging in the rendering of legal, financial, medical or professional advice. The content within this book has been derived from various sources. Please consult a licensed professional before attempting any techniques outlined in this book.

By reading this document, the reader agrees that under no circumstances is the author responsible for any losses, direct or indirect, which are incurred as a result of the use of information contained within this document, including, but not limited to, — errors, omissions, or inaccuracies.

TABLE OF CONTENTS

SMOOTHIES & BREAKFAST

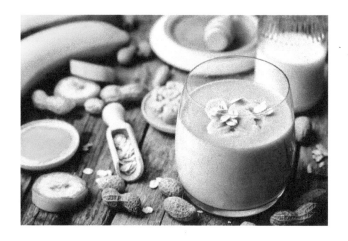

Curried Coconut Chicken

Preparation Time: 10 minutes

Cooking Time: 6 Hours Serve: 8

Ingredients:

- 6 chicken thighs
- 14.5 oz coconut milk
- ½ tbsp curry powder
- 3 garlic cloves, minced
- 1 onion, sliced
- 1 tbsp olive oil
- 2 green onion, sliced
- 3 tbsp fresh cilantro, chopped
- 3 cups chicken broth
- 1/4 tsp pepper
- 1 tsp salt

Directions:

1. Add oil into the crockpot.
2. Add all ingredients except green onion and cilantro into the crock pot and stir well.
3. Cover and cook on high for 6 hours.
4. Serve and enjoy.

Nutritional Value (Amount per Serving):

Calories 332

Fat 25 g

Carbohydrates 8 g

Sugar 3 g

Protein 24 g

Cholesterol 65 mg

Cheesy Garlic Bread Chaffle

Time: 15 minutes Serve: 2

Ingredients:

- 1 egg, lightly beaten

- 1 tsp parsley, minced

- 2 tbsp parmesan cheese, grated

- 1 tbsp butter, melted

- 1/4 tsp garlic powder

- 1/4 tsp baking powder, gluten-free

- 1 tsp coconut flour

- 1/2 cup cheddar cheese, shredded

Directions:

1. Preheat your waffle maker.

2. In a bowl, whisk egg, garlic powder, baking powder, coconut flour, and cheddar cheese until well combined.

3. Spray waffle maker with cooking spray.

4. Pour half of the batter in the hot waffle maker and cook for 3 minutes or until set. Repeat with the remaining batter.

5. Brush chaffles with melted butter.

6. Place chaffles on baking tray and top with parmesan cheese and broil until cheese melted.

7. Garnish with parsley and serve.

Nutrition: Calories 248 Fat 19.4 g
Carbohydrates 5.4 g Sugar 1 g

Keto Oreo Chaffles

Preparation Time: 13 minutes Cooking Time: 28 minutes Servings: 4

Ingredients:

For the Oreo chaffles:

- 2 eggs, beaten

- 1 cup finely grated mozzarella cheese

- 2 tbsp almond flour

- 1 tbsp unsweetened dark cocoa powder

- 2 tbsp erythritol

- 1 tbsp cream cheese, softened

- ½ tsp vanilla extract

For the glaze:

- 1 tbsp swerve confectioner's sugar

- 1 tsp water

Directions:

1. Preheat the waffle iron.

2. In a medium bowl, combine all the ingredients for the Oreo chaffles until adequately mixed.

3. Open the iron and pour in a quarter of the batter. Close the iron and cook until crispy, 7 minutes.

4. Remove the chaffle onto a plate and set aside.

5. Make 3 more chaffles with the remaining batter and transfer to a plate to cool.

For the glaze:

1. In a small bowl, whisk the swerve confectioner's sugar and water until smooth.

2. Drizzle a little of the glaze over each chaffle and serve after.

Nutrition: **Calories 50; Fats 3.64g;** Carbs 1.27g; Net Carbs 0.77g; Protein 3.4g

Fried Pickle Chaffle Sticks

Preparation Time: 10 minutes Cooking Time: 28 minutes Servings: 4

Ingredients:

- **1 egg, beaten**

- **¼ cup pork rinds**

- **½ cup finely grated mozzarella cheese**

- **½ tbsp pickle juice**

- **8 thin pickle slices, patted**
  with a paper towel

Directions:

1. Preheat the waffle iron.

2. In a medium bowl, combine the egg, pork rinds, mozzarella cheese, and pickle juice.

3. Open the iron and pour in 2 tbsp of the mixture, lay two pickle slices on top, and cover with 2 tbsp of the batter.

4. Close the iron and cook until brown and crispy, 7 minutes.

5. Remove the chaffle onto a plate and set aside.

6. Make 3 more chaffles in the same manner, using the remaining ingredients.

7. Cut the chaffles into sticks and serve after with cheese dip.

Nutrition: Calories 68; Fats 4.17g; Carbs 2.2g; Net Carbs 2.0g; Protein 5.25g

Keto Chaffle Churro Sticks

Preparation Time: 10 minutes Cooking Time: 28 minutes Servings: 4

Ingredients:

- 1 egg, beaten

- ½ cup finely grated mozzarella cheese

- 2 tbsp swerve brown sugar

- ½ tsp cinnamon powder

Directions:

1. Preheat the waffle iron.

2. Combine all the ingredients in a medium bowl until smooth.

3. Open the iron and pour in a quarter of the mixture. Close the iron and cook until golden brown and crispy, 7 minutes.

4. Remove the chaffle onto a plate and set aside.

5. Make 3 more chaffles with the remaining ingredients

6. Cut the chaffles into 4 sticks and serve after.

Nutrition: Calories 45; Fats 3.2g; Carbs 1.08g; Net Carbs 0.78g; Protein 2.95g

Cheeseburger Chaffle

Preparation Time: 15 minutes Cooking Time: 15 minutes Servings: 2

Ingredients:

- 1 lb. ground beef

- 1 onion, minced

- 1 tsp. parsley, chopped

- 1 egg, beaten

- Salt and pepper to taste

- 1 tablespoon olive oil

- 4 basic chaffles

- 2 lettuce leaves

- 2 cheese slices

- 1 tablespoon dill pickles

- Ketchup

- Mayonnaise

Directions:

1. In a large bowl, combine the ground beef, onion, parsley, egg, salt and pepper.

2. Mix well.

3. Form 2 thick patties.

4. Add olive oil to the pan.

5. Place the pan over medium heat.

6. Cook the patty for 3 to 5 minutes per side or until fully cooked.

7. Place the patty on top of each chaffle.

8. Top with lettuce, cheese and pickles.

9. Squirt ketchup and mayo over the patty and veggies.

10. 1Top with another chaffle.

Nutrition:

Calories 325 Total Fat 16.3g Saturated Fat 6.5g Cholesterol 157mg Sodium 208mg Total Carbohydrate 3g Dietary Fiber 0.7g Total Sugars 1.4g Protein 39.6g Potassium 532mg

Sausage Ball Chaffles

Preparation Time: 15 minutes Cooking Time: 28 minutes Servings: 4

Ingredients:

- 1 lb Italian sausage, crumbled

- 3 tbsp almond flour

- 2 tsp baking powder

- 1 egg, beaten

- ¼ cup finely grated Parmesan cheese

- 1 cup finely grated cheddar cheese

Directions:

1. Preheat the waffle iron.

2. Pour all the ingredients into a medium mixing bowl and mix well with your hands.

3. Open the iron, lightly grease with cooking spray and add 3 tbsp of the sausage mixture. Close the iron and cook for 4 minutes.

4. Open the iron, flip the chaffles and cook further for 3 minutes.

5. Remove the chaffle onto a plate and make 3 more using the rest of the mixture.

6. Cut each chaffle into sticks or quarters and enjoy after.

Nutrition: Calories 465; Fats 33.5g; Carbs 10.87g; Net Carbs 7.57g; Protein 32.52g

Garlic Bread Chaffles

Preparation Time: 10 minutes Cooking Time: 14 minutes Servings: 2

Ingredients:

- 1 egg, beaten

- ½ cup finely grated mozzarella cheese

- 1 tsp Italian seasoning

- ½ tsp garlic powder

- 1 tsp chive-flavored cream cheese

Directions:

1. Preheat the waffle iron.

2. Mix all the ingredients in a medium bowl until well combined.

3. Open the iron and add half of the mixture. Close and cook until golden brown and crispy, 7 minutes.

4. Remove the chaffle onto a plate and make a second one with the remaining batter.

5. Cut each chaffle into sticks or quarters and enjoy after.

Nutrition: Calories 51; Fats 3.56g; Carbs 1.57g; Net Carbs 1.27g; Protein 3.13g

Pumpkin-Cinnamon Churro Sticks

Preparation Time: 10 minutes Cooking Time: 14 minutes Servings: 2

Ingredients:

- **3 tbsp coconut flour**

- **¼ cup pumpkin puree**

- **1 egg, beaten**

- **½ cup finely grated mozzarella cheese**

- **2 tbsp sugar-free maple syrup** + more for serving

- **1 tsp baking powder**

- **1 tsp vanilla extract**

- **½ tsp pumpkin spice seasoning**
    - **1/8 tsp salt**

    - **1 tbsp cinnamon powder**

Directions:

1. Preheat the waffle iron.

2. Mix all the ingredients in a medium bowl until well combined.

3. Open the iron and add half of the mixture. Close and cook until golden brown and crispy, 7 minutes.

4. Remove the chaffle onto a plate and make 1 more with the remaining batter.

5. Cut each chaffle into sticks, drizzle the top with more maple syrup and serve after.

Nutrition: Calories 219; Fats 9.72g; Carbs 8.64g; Net Carbs 4.34g; Protein 25.27g

Crunchy Zucchini Chaffle

Time: 20 minutes Serve: 8

Ingredients:

- 2 eggs, lightly beaten
- 1 garlic clove, minced
- 1 1/2 tbsp onion, minced
- 1 cup cheddar cheese, grated
- 1 small zucchini, grated and squeeze out all liquid

Directions:

1. Preheat your waffle maker.

2. In a bowl, mix eggs, garlic, onion, zucchini, and cheese until well combined.

3. Spray waffle maker with cooking spray.

4. Pour 1/4 cup batter in the hot waffle maker and cook for 5 minutes or until golden brown. Repeat with the remaining batter.

5. Serve and enjoy.

Nutrition: Calories 76 Fat 5.8 g
Carbohydrates 1.1 g Sugar 0.5 g
Protein 5.1 g Cholesterol 56 mg

~
7
3
~

Guacamole Chaffle Bites

Preparation Time: 10 minutes Cooking Time: 14 minutes
Servings: 2

Ingredients:

- 1 large turnip, cooked and mashed

- 2 bacon slices, cooked and finely chopped

- ½ cup finely grated Monterey Jack cheese

- 1 egg, beaten

- 1 cup guacamole for topping

Directions:

1. Preheat the waffle iron.
2. Mix all the ingredients except for the guacamole in a medium bowl.

3. Open the iron and add half of the mixture. Close and cook for 4 minutes. Open the lid, flip the chaffle and cook further until golden brown and crispy, 3 minutes.

4. Remove the chaffle onto a plate and

make another in the same manner.

5. Cut each chaffle into wedges, top with the guacamole and serve afterward.

Nutrition: Calories 311; Fats 22.52g; Carbs 8.29g; Net Carbs 5.79g; Protein 13.62g

Baked Chicken Wings

Preparation Time: 10 minutes Cooking Time: 50 minutes

Serve: 4

Ingredients:

- 2 lbs chicken wings
- 1 tbsp lemon pepper seasoning
- 2 tbsp butter, melted
- 4 tbsp olive oil

Directions:

1. Preheat the oven to 400 F.
2. Toss chicken wings with olive oil.
3. Arrange chicken wings on a baking tray and bake for 50 minutes.
4. In a small bowl, mix together lemon pepper seasoning and butter.
5. Remove wings from oven and brush with butter and seasoning mixture.
6. Serve and enjoy.

Nutritional Value (Amount per Serving):

Calories 606

Fat 36 g

Carbohydrates 1 g

Sugar 0 g

Protein 65 g

Cholesterol 217 mg

Chicken with

Spinach Broccoli

Preparation Time: 10 minutes Cooking Time: 10 minutes Serve: 4

Ingredients:

- 1 lb chicken breasts, cut into pieces
- 4 oz cream cheese
- 1/2 cup parmesan cheese, shredded
- 2 cups baby spinach
- 2 cup broccoli florets
- 1 tomato, chopped
- 2 garlic cloves, minced
- 1 tsp Italian seasoning
- 2 tbsp olive oil
- Pepper
- Salt

Directions:

1. Heat oil in a saucepan over medium- high heat.
2. Add chicken, season with pepper, Italian seasoning, and salt and sauté for 5 minutes or until chicken cooked through.
3. Add garlic and sauté for a minute.
4. Add cream cheese, parmesan cheese, spinach, broccoli,

and tomato and cook for 3-4 minutes more.

5.   Serve and enjoy.

Nutritional Value (Amount per Serving):

Calories 444

Fat 28 g

Carbohydrates 5.9 g

Sugar 1.4 g

Protein 40 g

Cholesterol 140 mg

PORK, BEEF & LAMB RECIPES

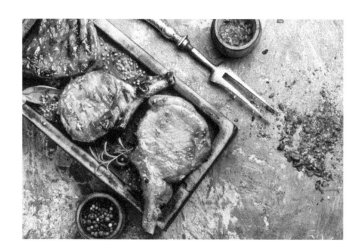

Herb Pork Chops

Preparation Time: 10 minutes Cooking Time: 30 minutes

Serve: 4

Ingredients:

- 4 pork chops, boneless
- 1 tbsp olive oil
- 2 garlic cloves, minced
- 1 tsp dried rosemary, crushed
- 1 tsp oregano
- ½ tsp thyme
- 1 tbsp fresh rosemary, chopped
- ¼ tsp pepper
- ¼ tsp salt

Directions:

1. Preheat the oven 425 F.
2. Season pork chops with pepper and salt and set aside.
3. In a small bowl, mix together garlic, oil, rosemary, oregano, thyme, and fresh rosemary and rub over pork chops.
4. Place pork chops on baking tray and roast for 10 minutes.
5. Turn heat to 350 F and roast for 25 minutes more.

6. Serve and enjoy.

Nutritional Value (Amount per Serving):

Calories 260

Fat 22 g

Carbohydrates 2.5 g

Sugar 0 g

Protein 19 g

Cholesterol 65 mg

SEAFOOD & FISH
RECIPES

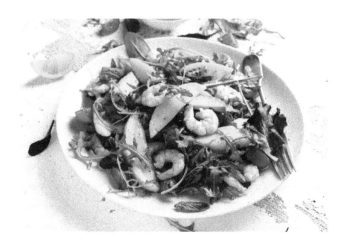

Roasted Green Beans

Preparation Time: 10 minutes Cooking Time: 25 minutes

Serve: 4

Ingredients:

- 1 lb frozen green beans
- ¼ tsp red pepper flakes
- 1/4 tsp garlic powder
- 2 tbsp olive oil
- 1/2 tsp onion powder
- 1/2 tsp pepper
- 1/2 tsp salt

Directions:

1. Preheat the oven to 425 F.
2. In a large bowl, add all ingredients and mix well.
3. Spread green beans baking tray and bake for 30 minutes.
4. Serve and enjoy.

Nutritional Value (Amount per Serving):

Calories 95

Fat 7 g

Carbohydrates 9 g

Sugar 2 g

Protein 2 g

Cholesterol 0 mg

MEATLESS
MEALS

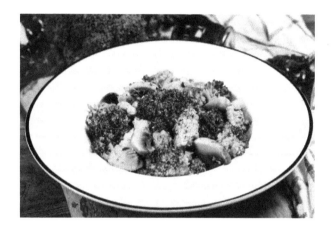

Delicious Pumpkin Risotto

Preparation Time: 10 minutes Cooking Time: 5 minutes Serve: 1

Ingredients:

- 1/4 cup pumpkin, grated
- 1 tbsp butter
- 1/2 cup water
- 1 cup cauliflower, grated
- 2 garlic cloves, chopped
- 1/8 tsp cinnamon
- Pepper
- Salt

Directions:

1. Melt butter in a pan over medium heat.
2. Add garlic, cauliflower, cinnamon and pumpkin into the pan and season with pepper and salt.
3. Cook until lightly softened. Add water and cook until done.
4. Serve and enjoy.

Nutritional Value (Amount per Serving):

Calories 155

Fat 11 g

Carbohydrates 11 g

Sugar 4.5 g

Protein 3.2 g

Cholesterol 30 mg

SOUPS, STEWS
& SALADS

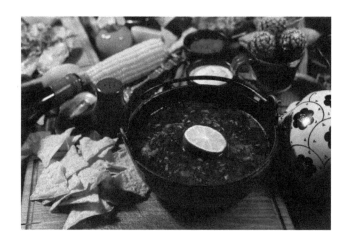

Creamy

Cauliflower Soup

Preparation Time: 10 minutes Cooking Time: 25 minutes

Serve: 4

Ingredients:

- 1/2 head cauliflower, chopped
- ½ tsp garlic powder
- ¼ cup onion, diced
- 1/4 tbsp olive oil
- 2 garlic cloves, minced
- 15 oz vegetable stock
- ¼ tsp pepper
- 1/2 tsp salt

Directions:

1. Heat olive oil in a saucepan over medium heat.
2. Add onion and garlic and sauté for 4 minutes.
3. Add cauliflower and stock and stir well. Bring to boil.
4. Cover pan with lid and simmer for 15 minutes.
5. Season with garlic powder, pepper, and salt.
6. Puree the soup using blender until smooth.
7. Serve and enjoy.

Nutritional Value (Amount per Serving):

Calories 41

Fat 2 g

Carbohydrates 4 g

Sugar 2 g

Protein 3 g

Cholesterol 0 mg

BRUNCH &
DINNER

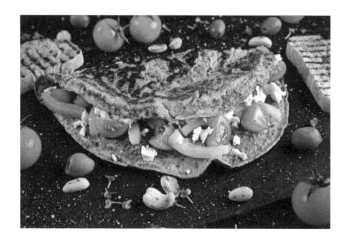

Protein Muffins

Preparation Time: 10 minutes Cooking Time: 15 minutes

Serve: 12

Ingredients:

- 8 eggs
- 2 scoop vanilla protein powder
- 8 oz cream cheese
- 4 tbsp butter, melted

Directions:

1. In a large bowl, combine together cream cheese and melted butter.
2. Add eggs and protein powder and whisk until well combined.
3. Pour batter into the greased muffin pan.
4. Bake at 350 F for 25 minutes.
5. Serve and enjoy.

Nutritional Value (Amount per Serving):

Calories 149

Fat 12 g

Carbohydrates 2 g

Sugar 0.4 g

Protein 8 g

Cholesterol 115 mg

Healthy Waffles

Preparation Time: 10 minutes Cooking Time:
10 minutes

Serve: 4

Ingredients:

- 8 drops liquid stevia
- 1/2 tsp baking soda
- 1 tbsp chia seeds
- 1/4 cup water
- 2 tbsp sunflower seed butter
- 1 tsp cinnamon
- 1 avocado, peel, pitted and mashed
- 1 tsp vanilla
- 1 tbsp lemon juice
- 3 tbsp coconut flour

Directions:

1. Preheat the waffle iron.
2. In a small bowl, add water and chia seeds and soak for 5 minutes.
3. Mash together sunflower seed butter, lemon juice, vanilla, stevia, chia mixture, and avocado.
4. Mix together cinnamon, baking soda, and coconut flour.
5. Add wet ingredients to the dry ingredients and

mix well.

6. Pour waffle mixture into the hot waffle iron and cook on each side for 3-5 minutes.

7. Serve and enjoy.

Nutritional Value (Amount per Serving):

Calories 220

Fat 17 g

Carbohydrates 13 g

Sugar 1.2 g

Protein 5.1 g

Cholesterol 0 mg

DESSERTS & DRINKS

Blackberry Pops

Preparation Time: 10 minutes Cooking Time:
10 minutes

Serve: 6

Ingredients:

- 1 tsp liquid stevia
- ½ cup water
- 1 fresh sage leaf
- 1 cup blackberries

Directions:

1. Add all ingredients into the blender and blend until smooth.
2. Pour blended mixture into the ice pop molds and place in refrigerator for overnight.
3. Serve and enjoy.

Nutritional Value (Amount per Serving):

Calories 10

Fat 0.1 g

Carbohydrates 2.3 g

Sugar 1.2 g

Protein 0.3 g

Cholesterol 0 mg

BREAKFAST RECIPES

Clementine and Pistachio Ricotta

Serves: 1

Prep Time: 10 mins

Ingredients

- 2 teaspoons pistachios, chopped
- ⅓ cup ricotta
- 2 strawberries
- 1 tablespoon butter, melted
- 1 clementine, peeled and segmented

Directions

1. Put the ricotta into a serving bowl.
2. Top with clementine segments, strawberries, pistachios and butter to serve.

Nutrition Amount per serving

Calories 311

Total Fat 25.1g 32% Saturated Fat 15.1g 76%

Cholesterol 71mg 24%

Sodium 243mg 11%

Total Carbohydrate 12.7g 5% Dietary Fiber 1.2g 4%

Total Sugars 7.1g Protein 10.7g

APPETIZERS & DESSERTS

Roasted Spicy Garlic Eggplant Slices

Serves: 4

Prep Time: 35 mins

Ingredients

- 2 tablespoons olive oil
- 1 eggplant, sliced into rounds
- 1 teaspoon garlic powder
- Salt and red pepper
- ½ teaspoon Italian seasoning

Directions

1. Preheat the oven to 4000F and line a baking sheet with parchment paper.
2. Arrange the eggplant slices on a baking sheet and drizzle with olive oil.
3. Season with Italian seasoning, garlic powder, salt and red pepper.
4. Transfer to the oven and bake for about 25 minutes.
5. Remove from the oven and serve hot.

Nutrition Amount per serving

Calories 123

Total Fat 9.7g 12%

Saturated Fat 1.4g

7% Cholesterol 0mg

0%

Sodium 3mg 0%

Total Carbohydrate

10g 4% Dietary Fiber

5.6g 20% Total Sugars

4.9g

Protein 1.7g

PORK & BEEF RECIPES

Pork with Butternut Squash Stew

Serves: 4

Prep Time: 40 mins

Ingredients

½ pound butternut squash, peeled and cubed

- 1 pound lean pork
- 2 tablespoons butter
- Salt and black pepper, to taste
- 1 cup beef stock

Directions

- Put the butter and lean pork in a skillet and cook for about 5 minutes.
- Add butternut squash, beef stock and season with salt and black pepper.
- Cover with lid and cook for about 25 minutes on medium low heat.
- Dish out to a bowl and serve hot.

Nutrition Amount per serving

Calories 319

Total Fat 17.1g 22% Saturated Fat 7.9g

39% Cholesterol 105mg 35%

Sodium 311mg 14%

Total Carbohydrate 6.7g 2% Dietary

Fiber 1.1g 4%

Total Sugars 1.3g Protein 33.7g

SEAFOOD RECIPES

Garlicky Lemon Scallops

Serves: 6

Prep Time: 30 mins

Ingredients

- 2 pounds scallops
- 3 garlic cloves, minced
- 5 tablespoons butter, divided
- Red pepper flakes, kosher salt and black pepper
- 1 lemon, zest and juice

Directions

1. Heat 2 tablespoons butter over medium heat in a large skillet and add scallops, kosher salt and black pepper.
2. Cook for about 5 minutes per side until golden and transfer to a plate.
3. Heat remaining butter in a skillet and add garlic and red pepper flakes.
4. Cook for about 1 minute and stir in lemon juice and zest.

5. Return the scallops to the skillet and stir well.

6. Dish out on a platter and serve hot.

Nutrition Amount per serving

Calories 224

Total Fat 10.8g 14% Saturated Fat 6.2g 31% Cholesterol 75mg 25%

Sodium 312mg 14%

Total Carbohydrate 5.2g 2% Dietary Fiber 0.4g 1%

Total Sugars 0.3g Protein 25.7g

Lemon Cream Bok Choy

Serves: 4

Prep Time: 45 mins Ingredients

- 28 oz. bok choy

- 1 large lemon, juice and zest

- ¾ cup heavy whipping cream

- 1 cup parmesan cheese, freshly grated

- 1 teaspoon black pepper

Directions

1. Preheat the oven to 3500F and lightly grease a baking dish.
2. Pour the cream over the bok choy evenly and drizzle with the lemon juice.
3. Mix well and transfer to the baking dish.
4. Top with parmesan cheese, lemon zest and black pepper and place in the oven.
5. Bake for about 30 minutes until lightly browned and remove from the oven to serve hot.

Nutrition Amount per serving

Calories 199

Total Fat 14.8g 19% Saturated Fat 9.3g 46%

Cholesterol 51mg 17%

Sodium 398mg 17%

Total Carbohydrate 7.7g 3%
Dietary Fiber 2.5g 9% Total Sugars 2.7g

Protein 12.7g

Butter Fried Green Cabbage

Serves: 4

Prep Time: 30 mins Ingredients

- 3 oz. butter

- Salt and black pepper, to taste

- 25 oz. green cabbage, shredded

- 1 tablespoon basil

- ¼ teaspoon red chili flakes

Directions

1. Heat butter in a large skillet over medium heat and add cabbage.
2. Sauté for about 15 minutes, stirring occasionally, until the cabbage is golden brown.
3. Stir in basil, red chili flakes, salt and black pepper and cook for about 3 minutes.
4. Dish out to a bowl and serve hot.

Nutrition Amount per serving

Calories 197

Total Fat 17.4g 22% Saturated Fat 11g 55% Cholesterol 46mg 15%

Sodium 301mg 13%

Total Carbohydrate 10.3g 4%

Dietary Fiber 4.5g 16%
   Total Sugars 5.7gProtein 2.5g

Broccoli and Cheese

Serves: 4

Prep Time: 20 mins

Ingredients

- 5½ oz. cheddar cheese, shredded

- 23 oz. broccoli, chopped

- 2 oz. butter

- Salt and black pepper, to taste

- 4 tablespoons sour cream

Directions

1. Heat butter in a large skillet over medium high heat and add broccoli, salt and black pepper.
2. Cook for about 5 minutes and stir in the sour cream and cheddar cheese.
3. Cover with lid and cook for about 8 minutes on medium low heat.
4. Dish out to a bowl and serve hot.

Nutrition Amount per serving

Calories 340

Total Fat 27.5g 35% Saturated Fat 17.1g 85%

Cholesterol 77mg 26%

Sodium 384mg 17%
Total Carbohydrate 11.9g 4%

Dietary Fiber 4.3g 15% Total Sugars 3g Protein 14.8g

Broccoli Gratin

Serves: 4

Prep Time: 35 mins Ingredients

- 2 oz. salted butter, for frying

- 5 oz. parmesan cheese, shredded

- 20 oz. broccoli, in florets

- 2 tablespoons Dijon mustard

- ¾ cup crème fraiche

Directions

1. Preheat the oven to 4000F and grease a baking dish lightly.
2. Heat half the butter in a pan on medium low heat and add chopped broccoli.
3. Sauté for about 5 minutes and transfer to the baking dish.
4. Mix the rest of the butter with Dijon mustard and crème fraiche.
5. Pour this mixture in the baking dish and top with parmesan cheese.
6. Transfer to the oven and bake for about 18 minutes.
7. Dish out to a bowl and serve hot.

Nutrition Amount per serving Calories 338

Total Fat 27.4g 35% Saturated Fat 12.4g 62% Cholesterol 56mg 19%

Sodium 546mg 24%

Total Carbohydrate 11.1g 4%

Dietary Fiber 4g 14% Total Sugars 2.5g Protein 16.2g

Lemon Cream Bok Choy

Serves: 4

Prep Time: 45 mins

Ingredients

- 28 oz. bok choy
- 1 large lemon, juice and zest
- ¾ cup heavy whipping cream
- 1 cup parmesan cheese, freshly grated
- 1 teaspoon black pepper

Directions

1. Preheat the oven to 3500F and lightly grease a baking dish.
2. Pour the cream over the bok choy evenly and drizzle with the lemon juice.
3. Mix well and transfer to the baking Sodium 301mg 13% *Vegan And Vegetarian* dish.
4. Top with parmesan cheese, lemon zest and black pepper and place in the oven.
5. Bake for about 30 minutes until lightly browned and remove from the oven to serve hot.

Nutrition Amount per serving

Calories 199

Total Fat 14.8g 19% Saturated Fat 9.3g 46%

Cholesterol 51mg 17%

Sodium 398mg 17%

Total Carbohydrate 7.7g 3% Dietary Fiber 2.5g 9%

Total Sugars 2.7g Protein 12.7g

CHICKEN AND POULTRY RECIPES

Low Carb Chicken Nuggets

Serves: 6

Prep Time: 25 mins

Ingredients

- ¼ cup mayonnaise
- 2 medium chicken breasts
- 1 cup blanched almond flour
- 2 tablespoons olive oil
- Sea salt and black pepper, to taste

Directions

1. Put the chicken in the salted water for about 10 minutes.
2. Drain it and cut the chicken into nugget sized pieces.
3. Put mayonnaise in one bowl and mix almond flour, sea salt and black pepper in another bowl.
4. Coat each chicken nugget with mayonnaise and dredge in the almond flour mixture.

5. Heat oil over medium high heat in a skillet and add chicken nuggets in a single layer.

6. Cook for about 3 minutes per side until golden and dish out to serve.

Nutrition Amount per serving

Calories 283

Total Fat 20.4g 26% Saturated Fat 2.8g 14%

Cholesterol 46mg 15%

Sodium 118mg   5%

Total Carbohydrate 6.3g 2% Dietary Fiber 2g 7%

Total Sugars 0.6g Protein 18.2g

BREAKFAST RECIPES

Cinnamon Coconut Pancake

Total Time: 15 minutes

Serves: 1

Ingredients:

- 1/2 cup almond milk
- 1/4 cup coconut flour
- 2 tbsp egg replacer
- 8 tbsp water
- 1 packet stevia
- 1/8 tsp cinnamon
- 1/2 tsp baking powder
- 1 tsp vanilla extract
- 1/8 tsp salt

Directions:

1. In a small bowl, mix together egg replacer and 8 tablespoons of water.
2. Add all ingredients into the mixing bowl and stir until combined.
3. Spray pan with cooking spray and heat over medium heat.

4. Pour the desired amount of batter onto hot pan and cook until lightly golden brown.

5. Flip pancake and cook for a few minutes more.

6. Serve and enjoy.

Nutritional Value (Amount per Serving): Calories 110; Fat 4.3 g; Carbohydrates 10.9 g; Sugar 2.8 g; Protein 7 g; Cholesterol 0 mg;

Zucchini Muffins

Total Time: 35 minutes Serves: 8

Ingredients:

- 1 cup almond flour
- 1 zucchini, grated
- 1/4 cup coconut oil, melted
- 15 drops liquid stevia
- 1/2 tsp baking soda
- 1/2 cup coconut flour
- 1/2 cup walnut, chopped
- 1 1/2 tsp cinnamon
- 3/4 cup unsweetened applesauce
- 1/8 tsp salt

Directions:

1. Preheat the oven to 325 F/ 162 C.
2. Spray muffin tray with cooking spray and set aside.
3. In a bowl, combine together grated zucchini, coconut oil, and stevia.
4. In another bowl, mix together coconut flour, baking soda, almond flour, walnut, cinnamon, and salt.
5. Add zucchini mixture into the coconut flour mixture and mix well.
6. Add applesauce and stir until well combined.
7. Pour batter into the prepared muffin tray and bake in

preheated oven for 25-30 minutes.

8. Serve and enjoy.

Nutritional Value (Amount per Serving): Calories 229; Fat 18.9 g; Carbohydrates 12.5 g; Sugar 3.4 g; Protein 5.2 g; Cholesterol 0 mg;

LUNCH RECIPES

Tomato Pumpkin Soup

Total Time: 25 minutes Serves: 4

Ingredients:

- 2 cups pumpkin, diced
- 1/2 cup tomato, chopped
- 1/2 cup onion, chopped
- 1 1/2 tsp curry powder
- 1/2 tsp paprika
- 2 cups vegetable stock
- 1 tsp olive oil
- 1/2 tsp garlic, minced

Directions:

- ➢ In a saucepan, add oil, garlic, and onion and sauté for 3 minutes over medium heat.
- ➢ Add remaining ingredients into the saucepan and bring to boil.
- ➢ Reduce heat and cover and simmer for 10 minutes.
- ➢ Puree the soup using a blender until smooth.
- ➢ Stir well and serve warm.

Nutritional Value (Amount per Serving): Calories 70; Fat 2.7 g; Carbohydrates 13.8g; Sugar 6.3 g; Protein 1.9 g; Cholesterol 0 mg;

DINNER RECIPES

Baked Cauliflower

Total Time: 55 minutes Serves: 2

Ingredients:

- 1/2 cauliflower head, cut into florets
- 2 tbsp olive oil
- For seasoning:
- 1/2 tsp garlic powder
- 1/2 tsp ground cumin
- 1/2 tsp black pepper
- 1/2 tsp white pepper
- 1 tsp onion powder
- 1/4 tsp dried oregano
- 1/4 tsp dried basil
- 1/4 tsp dried thyme
- 1 tbsp ground cayenne pepper
- 2 tbsp ground paprika
- 2 tsp salt

Directions:

1. Preheat the oven to 400 F/ 200 C.
2. Spray a baking tray with cooking spray and set aside.

3. In a large bowl, mix together all seasoning ingredients.

4. Add oil and stir well. Add cauliflower to the bowl seasoning mixture and stir well to coat.

5. Spread the cauliflower florets on a baking tray and bake in preheated oven for 45 minutes.

6. Serve and enjoy.

Nutritional Value (Amount per Serving): Calories 177; Fat 15.6 g; Carbohydrates 11.5 g; Sugar 3.2 g; Protein 3.1 g; Cholesterol 0 mg;

DESSERT RECIPES

Chocolate Fudge

Total Time: 10 minutes Serves: 12

Ingredients:

4 oz unsweetened dark chocolate

- 3/4 cup coconut butter
- 15 drops liquid stevia
- 1 tsp vanilla extract

Directions:

1. Melt coconut butter and dark chocolate.
2. Add ingredients to the large bowl and combine well.
3. Pour mixture into a silicone loaf pan and place in refrigerator until set.
4. Cut into pieces and serve.

Nutritional Value (Amount per Serving): Calories 157; Fat 14.1 g; Carbohydrates 6.1 g; Sugar 1 g; Protein 2.3 g; Cholesterol 0 mg;

BREAKFAST RECIPES

Tuna Omelet

Breakfast would not be complete without a healthy omelet to get your day started on the right foot.

Total Prep & Cooking Time: 15 minutes

Level: Beginner Makes: 2 Omelets

Protein: 28 grams Net Carbs: 4.9 grams

Fat: 18 grams

Sugar: 1 gram

Calories: 260

What you need:

- 2 tbs coconut oil
- 1 medium green bell pepper, deseeded and diced
- 2 1/2 oz. canned tuna, spring water and drained
- 1/4 tsp salt
- 6 large eggs
- 1/8 tsp pepper

Steps:

1. Melt the coconut oil in a small skillet and fry the green pepper for approximately 3 minutes. Remove from the burner.

2. Transfer the peppers into a dish and combine the tuna until fully together. Set to the side.

3. Beat the eggs, salt, and pepper in a separate dish as the coconut oil is melting in a small non-stick skillet.

4. Move the pan around to ensure the entire base is coated in oil and very hot.

5. Empty the beaten eggs into the skillet and use a rubber spatula to lift the

   edge of the cooked eggs in several areas to allow the uncooked eggs to heat.

6. Once there is a thin layer of cooked egg created, leave the pan on the heat for half a minute to fully set.

7. Scoop half of the peppers and tuna onto one side of the eggs. Use the rubber spatula to flip over the cooked eggs to create an omelet.

8. Press down lightly until the omelet naturally seals and after approximately 1 minute, move to a serving plate.

9. Repeat steps 4 through 8 with the second omelet.

Baking Tip:

If you do not have a ton of time in the mornings, you can create the omelet filling the evening before and refrigerate in a lidded container.

Variation Tip:

You may choose to garnish the top of the omelet with additional salt and pepper to taste or chopped chives.

SNACK RECIPES

Spicy Deviled Eggs

This classic recipe that is a staple for any picnic or party has a kick that your taste buds will appreciate.

Total Prep & Cooking Time: 30 minutes Level: Beginner

Makes: 4 Helpings

Protein: 6 grams

Net Carbs: 1.5 grams Fat: 7 grams

Sugar: 1 gram

Calories: 94

What you need:

- 1/4 tsp cayenne pepper
- 2 large eggs, hardboiled
- 1/8 tsp cajun seasoning
- 4 thin slices of andouille sausage
- 1 tsp mustard
- 2 tsp mayonnaise, sugar-free
- 1/8 cup sauerkraut
- 1/4 tsp paprika

Steps:

1. Fill a small saucepan with 2 cups of the cold water to cover the eggs.

2. When the water begins to boil, set the timer for 7 minutes.

3. After the timer goes off, drain the water and cover the eggs with the remaining 2 cups of cold water.

4. Brown the sausage in a non-stick skillet until crispy. Remove to a platter covered in paper towels.

5. Peel and slice the eggs in halves long ways and transfer the yolks into a dish.

6. Combine the mayonnaise, cayenne pepper, Cajun seasoning, and mustard until smooth.

7. Place a slice of the sausage into the center of each egg and spoon the mixture on top of each.

8. Dust the top with paprika and serve.

DINNER RECIPES

Chicken Zucchini Meatballs

When you want an easy dinner, these meatballs will be quick to make after a hard

day at work.

Total Prep & Cooking Time: 25 minutes

Level: Beginner

Makes: 4 Helpings

Protein: 26 grams Net Carbs: 2.4 grams Fat:

4 grams

Sugar: 1 gram

Calories: 161

What you need:

- 16 oz. chicken breasts, boneless
- 1/2 tsp celery seeds
- 2 cups zucchini, chopped
- 1 large egg
- 2 cloves garlic, peeled
- 1/2 tbs salt
- 3 tsp oregano
- 1/2 tsp pepper

- 2 tbs coconut oil

Steps:

2. Set the temperature of the stove to heat at 180° Fahrenheit. Layer a flat sheet with baking lining and set aside.

3. Use a food blender pulse all the components for approximately 3 minutes until totally incorporated.

4. Dissolve the coconut oil in a non-stick skillet.

5. Scoop out the meat and hand roll into one-inch meatballs.

6. Transfer to the hot oil and brown on each side for approximately 2 minutes.

7. Spoon the meatballs onto the prepped sheet and heat for about 10 minutes.

8. Serve warm and enjoy!

UNUSUAL DELICIOUS MEAL RECIPES

Mediterranean

Lamb Chops

Get a taste of the Mediterranean with this

unique mix of spices that will really make your mouth water.
Total Prep & Cooking Time: 20 minutes

Level: Beginner

Makes: 4 Helpings (2 Chops per serving) Protein: 29 grams

Net Carbs: 1 gram Fat: 8 grams

Sugar: 1 gram

Calories: 164

What you need:

- 2 tsp lemon juice
- 1/4 tsp pepper
- 14 oz. lamb loin chops, trimmed and bone in
- 1/2 tsp extra virgin olive oil
- 2/3 tsp salt
- 1 1/2 cloves garlic, crushed
- 2 tsp Za'atar

Steps:

1. Heat the grill to the temperature of 350° Fahrenheit.
2. Prepare the lamb chops by brushing with garlic and oil.
3. Sprinkle the lemon juice over each side and dust with the salt, Za'atar, and pepper.
4. Grill on each side for approximately 4 minutes until your desired crispiness.

Baking Tip:

Alternatively, you can broil in the stove for about 5 minutes on each side.

If Za'atar seasoning is not available, you can easily make your own.

You need the following ingredients:

- 1/3 tbs oregano seasoning
- 1/8 tsp sea salt
- 1/3 tbs marjoram
- 1/8 tbs roasted sesame seeds
- 1/3 tbs thyme
- 3 tbs sumac

Peanut Stew

Coming all the way from Africa, this is a popular dish that is filled with fats that will help keep you in ketosis.

Total Prep & Cooking Time: 25 minutes

Level: Beginner

Makes: 4 Helpings

Protein: 14 grams Net Carbs: 6 grams Fat: 26 grams

Sugar: 0 grams

Calories: 286

What you need:

For the stew:

- 16 oz. tofu, extra firm and cubed
- 1/4 tsp salt
- 3 tbs coconut oil
- 1/8 tsp pepper
- 3 tsp onion powder
- 1/2 tbs ginger, chopped finely

For the sauce:

- 4 tbs peanut butter
- 8 oz. vegetable broth, warmed
- 1/2 tsp turmeric
- 3 tsp sriracha
- 1 tsp paprika powder
- 4 oz. tomatoes, crushed

- 1/2 tsp cumin

Steps:

1. Heat the broth in a saucepan over medium heat. When boiling, remove from the burner.

2. Blend the sriracha, tomato sauce, cumin, turmeric, hot broth, peanut butter and paprika in the glass dish and integrate completely. It should thicken into a sauce. Set to the side.

3. Use a non-stick skillet to dissolve 2 tablespoons of coconut oil.

4. When the pan is hot, empty the cubes of tofu and brown on all sides taking approximately 4 minutes. Remove from the burner and transfer to a glass dish.

5. Combine the ginger, onion powder and the remaining tablespoon of coconut oil into the skillet and heat for 3 minutes.

6. Empty the browned tofu back into the skillet and continue to brown for an additional 2 minutes. Distribute into a serving bowl.

7. Dispense the sauce over the browned tofu and serve immediately.

Variation Tip:

You can garnish this meal with a half a cup of dry roasted peanuts if you prefer more peanut taste.

KETO DESSERTS RECIPES

Blueberry Bars

Serves: 4

Preparation time: 10 minutes Cooking time: 75 minutes

Ingredients:

- ¼ cup blueberries
- 1 tsp vanilla
- 1 tsp fresh lemon juice
- 2 tbsp erythritol
- ¼ cup almonds, sliced
- ¼ cup coconut flakes
- 3 tbsp coconut oil
- 2 tbsp coconut flour
- ½ cup almond flour
- 3 tbsp water
- 1 tbsp chia seeds

Directions:

1. Preheat the oven to 300 F/ 150 C.
2. Line baking dish with parchment paper and set aside.
3. In a small bowl, mix together water and chia seeds. Set aside.
4. In a bowl, combine together all ingredients. Add chia mixture

and stir well.

5. Pour mixture into the prepared baking dish and spread evenly.

6. Bake for 50 minutes. Remove from oven and allow to cool completely.

7. Cut into bars and serve.

Per Serving: Net Carbs: 2.8g; Calories: 136; Total Fat: 11.9g; Saturated Fat: 6.1g

Protein: 3.1g; Carbs: 5.5g; Fiber: 2.7g; Sugar: 1.3g; Fat 81% / Protein 10% / Carbs 9%

CAKE

Coconut Pie

Serves: 8

Preparation time: 10 minutes Cooking time: 20

minutes

Ingredients:

- 2 oz shredded coconut
- 1/4 cup erythritol
    - 1/4 cup coconut oil
    - oz coconut flakes
    - 1 tsp xanthan gum
    - 3/4 cup erythritol
    - 2 cups heavy cream

Directions:

1. Add coconut flakes, erythritol, and coconut oil into the food processor and process for 30-40 seconds.
2. Transfer coconut flakes mixed into the pie pan and spread evenly.
3. Lightly press down the mixture and bake at 350 F/ 180 C for 10 minutes.
4. Heat heavy cream in a saucepan over low heat.
5. Whisk in shredded coconut, powdered erythritol, and xanthan gum. Bring to boil.

6. Remove from heat and set aside to cool for 10 minutes.

7. Pour filling mixture onto the crust and place in the refrigerator for overnight.

8. Slice and serve.

Per Serving: Net Carbs: 2.5g; Calories: 206; Total Fat: 21.4g; Saturated Fat: 15.9g

Protein: 1.1g; Carbs: 3.8g; Fiber: 1.3g; Sugar: 1.7g; Fat 93% / Protein 3% / Carbs 4%

Quick & Simple

Strawberry Tart

Serves: 10

Preparation time: 10 minutes Cooking time: 22 minutes

Ingredients:

- 5 egg whites
- ½ cup butter, melted
- 1 tsp baking powder
- 1 tsp vanilla
- 1 lemon zest, grated
- 1 ½ cup almond flour
- 1/3 cup xylitol

Directions:

1. Preheat the oven to 375 F/ 190 C.
2. Spray the tart pan with cooking spray and set aside.
3. In a bowl, whisk egg whites until foamy.
4. Add sweetener and whisk until soft peaks form.
5. Add remaining ingredients except for strawberries and fold until well combined.
6. Pour mixture into the prepared tart pan and top with sliced strawberries.
7. Bake in preheated oven for 20-22 minutes.
8. Serve and enjoy.

Per Serving: Net Carbs: 3.9g; Calories: 195; Total Fat: 17.7g; Saturated Fat: 6.4g

Protein: 5.6g; Carbs: 5.9g; Fiber: 2g; Sugar: 0.9g; Fat 81% / Protein 11% / Carbs 8%

Delicious Custard Tarts

Serves: 8

Preparation time: 10 minutes Cooking time: 30 minutes

For crust:

- ¾ cup coconut flour

- 1 tbsp swerve

- 2 eggs

- ½ cup of coconut oil

- Pinch of salt

- For custard:

- 3 eggs

- ½ tsp nutmeg

- 5 tbsp swerve

- 1 ½ tsp vanilla

- 1 ¼ cup unsweetened almond milk

Directions:

1. For the crust: Preheat the oven to 400 F/ 200 C.
2. In a bowl, beat eggs, coconut oil, sweetener, and salt.
3. Add coconut flour and mix until dough is formed.
4. Add dough in the tart pan and spread evenly.
5. Prick dough with a knife.
6. Bake in preheated oven for 10 minutes.
7. For the custard: Heat almond milk and vanilla in a

small pot until simmering.

8. Whisk together eggs and sweetener in a bowl. Slowly add almond milk and whisk constantly.

9. Strain custard well and pour into baked tart base.

10. Bake in the oven at 300 F for 30 minutes.

11. Sprinkle nutmeg on top and serve.

Per Serving: Net Carbs: 2.2g; Calories: 175; Total Fat: 17.2g; Saturated Fat: 12.9g

Protein: 3.8g; Carbs: 2.9g; Fiber: 0.7g; Sugar: 0.4g; Fat 87% / Protein 8% / Carbs 5%

CANDY: BEGINNER

Mascarpone

Cheese Candy

Serves: 10

Preparation time: 5 minutes Cooking time: 5
minutes

Ingredients:

- 1 cup mascarpone cheese, softened
- 1/4 cup pistachios, chopped
- 3 tbsp swerve
- 1/2 tsp vanilla

Directions:

1. In a small bowl, add swerve, vanilla, and mascarpone
   and mix together until smooth.
2. Place chopped pistachios in a small shallow dish.
3. Make small balls from cheese mixture and roll in
   chopped pistachios.
   4. Refrigerate for 1 hour.
   5. Serve and enjoy.

Per Serving: Net Carbs: 1.6g; Calories: 53 Total Fat: 3.9g; Saturated Fat: 2.1 Protein: 3.1g; Carbs: 1.8g; Fiber: 0.2g; Sugar: 0.2g; Fat 66% / Protein 23% / Carbs 11%

COOKIES: BEGINNER

Intermediate:

CocoNut Almond Cookies

Serves: 40

Preparation time: 5 minutes Cooking time: 10 minutes

Ingredients:

- 3 cups unsweetened shredded coconut
- 3/4 cup erythritol
- 1 cup almond flour
- 1/4 cup can coconut milk

Directions:

1. Spray a baking sheet with cooking spray and set aside.
2. Add all ingredients to a large bowl and mix until combined.
3. Make small balls from mixture and place on a prepared baking sheet and press lightly into a cookie shape.
4. Place in refrigerator until firm.
5. Serve and enjoy.

Per Serving: Net Carbs: 0.9g; Calories: 71 Total Fat: 6.3g; Saturated Fat: 4.4g

Protein: 1.2g; Carbs: 2.4g; Fiber: 1.5g; Sugar: 0.7g; Fat 85% / Protein 9% / Carbs 6%

FROZEN DESSERT: BEGINNER

Cinnamon Ice Cream

Serves: 8

Preparation time: 10 minutes Cooking time: 30 minutes

Ingredients:

- 1 egg yolk
- ½ tsp vanilla
- 3 tsp cinnamon
- ¾ cup erythritol
- 2 cups heavy whipping cream
- Pinch of salt

Directions:

1. Add all ingredients to the mixing bowl and blend until well combined.
2. Pour ice cream mixture into the ice cream maker and churn ice cream according to the machine instructions.
3. Serve and enjoy.

Per Serving: Net Carbs: 1.1g; Calories: 113 Total Fat: 11.7g; Saturated Fat: 7.1g

Protein: 1g; Carbs: 1.6g; Fiber: 0.5g; Sugar: 0.1g; Fat 93% / Protein 3% / Carbs 4%

Expert: Classic Citrus Custard

Serves: 4

Preparation time: 10 minutes Cooking time: 10 minutes

Ingredients:

- 2 ½ cups heavy whipping cream
- ½ tsp orange extract
- 2 tbsp fresh lime juice
- ¼ cup fresh lemon juice
- ½ cup Swerve
- Pinch of salt

Directions:

1. Boil heavy whipping cream and sweetener in a saucepan for 5-6

minutes. Stir continuously.

2. Remove saucepan from heat and add orange extract, lime juice, lemon juice, and salt and mix well.
3. Pour custard mixture into ramekins.
4. Place ramekins in refrigerator for 6 hours.
5. Serve chilled and enjoy.

Per Serving: Net Carbs: 2.7g; Calories: 265; Total Fat: 27.9g; Saturated Fat: 17.4g

Protein: 1.7g; Carbs: 2.8g; Fiber: 0.1g; Sugar: 0.5g; Fat 94% / Protein 2% / Carbs 4%

BREAKFAST RECIPES

Pasta with Sausage and Broccoli Rabe

All out: 50 min Prep: 10 min

Idle: 15 min

Cook: 25 min

Yield: 8 servings

Ingredients

- 1 pound broccoli rabe, cut of harmed leaves

- 2 tablespoons water

- 1/2 pound Italian frankfurter, cut into quarter-inch cuts

- Salt

- 1 cup coarse, prepared bread morsels, toasted, discretionary trimming

- 1 pound orecchiette or other pasta noodle

- Pecorino Romano or Parmesan, discretionary enhancement

- 4 to 5 cloves garlic, meagerly cut

Direction

1. Cut the broccoli rabe into 3 to 4 inch pieces, disposing of the

stems. In an enormous pot of quickly bubbling water, whiten the broccoli rabe until delicate and cooked through, around 5 to 6 minutes. Before you channel broccoli rabe, save 1 cup of cooking fluid. Channel and wash the broccoli rabe with virus water until it has chilled. Spread it out on a towel to get done with depleting.

2. Then, cook the pasta in a huge pot of bubbling water as indicated by bundle

    headings until still somewhat firm.

3. While the pasta is cooking, place 2 tablespoons of water into a cool skillet with garlic and hotdog and after that go warmth to medium-low. Cook, blending once in a while, until garlic is brilliant and wiener is cooked through, around 5 to 7 minutes. Empty held broccoli water into container with frankfurter.

4. At the point when the pasta is cooked, channel it and spot back in pot you cooked it in and season with salt. Pour hotdog sauce over pasta and blend in cooked broccoli rabe. Taste and change seasonings. Serve right away.

5. In the event that the Queen's coming to supper: Garnish with crisp bread morsels or potentially newly ground pecorino Romano or parmesan cheddar

LUNCH RECIPES

Pumpkin Pie

Preparation Time: 8 hours Servings:8

Nutritional Values:

Fat: 29 g.

Protein: 7 g.

Carbs: 9 g.

Ingredients:

For the Crust

- 1 cup Walnuts, chopped
- 1 cup Almond Flour
- ¼ cup Erythritol
- 1/3 cup Melted Butter

For the Filling

- 1 14-oz can Pumpkin Puree
- ½ cup Erythritol
- 1 cup Heavy Cream
- 6 Egg Yolks
- 1 tbsp Gelatin
- 1 tsp Vanilla Extract
- 1 tsp Cinnamon Powder
- ¼ tsp Ground Ginger

- ¼ tsp Ground Nutmeg
- ¼ tsp Ground Cloves

Directions:

- Mix well. Pack the mixture into a 9- inch springform pan.
- Combine all ingredients for the filling in a pot. Whisk over medium heat until mixture starts to thicken.
- Pour filling into the crust and refrigerate overnight.

Keto Cheeseburger Muffin

Cooking time: 23 min Yield: 9 muffins

Nutrition facts: 96 calories per muffin: Carbs 3.7g, fats 7g, and proteins 3.9g.

Ingredients:

- 8 tbsp almond flour
- 8 tbsp flaxseed meal
- 1 tsp baking powder
- ½ tspsalt
- ¼ tsp pepper
- 2 eggs
- 4 tbsp sour cream

Hamburger Filling:

- 1 lb ground beef
- 2 tbsp tomato paste
- Salt, pepper,onion powder,garlic powder to taste

Toppings:

- oz cheddar cheese
- 1 pickle, sliced
- 2 tbsp ketchup
- 2 tbsp mustard

Steps:

1. Heat the oven to 175 C.
2. Combine together: ground beef+seasoning+salt+pepper. Fry
3. Mix together the dry ingredients: almond flour+flaxseed meal+baking powder+salt+pepper.
4. Put there:sour cream+eggs
5. Place the dough into the baking silicone cups, greased. Leave some space at the top.
6. Put the ground beef on the top of the dough.
7. Bake for 20 min.
8. Take out of the oven and place the cheese on the ground beef. Bake for 3 min more.
9. Put the topping and enjoy.

SNACKS RECIPES

Nuts buns with cheese

Servings: 6-8

Cooking time: 35 minutes

Nutrients per one serving: Calories: 102 | Fats: 14.1 g | Carbs: 2.6 g | Proteins: 20 g

Ingredients:

- ½ cup almond flour
- ¼ cup sesame seeds
- ¼ cup sunflower seeds
- 1 tbsp psyllium
- 3 eggs
- 1 ½ cup grated cheese
- 1 tsp baking powder

Cooking process:

1. The oven to be preheated to 200°C (400°F).
2. In a bowl, beat the eggs by a mixer until dense mass. Add cheese and dry ingredients, mix well. Leave the dough for 10 minutes.
3. Cover the baking sheet with parchment. Make the small buns and lay out them on a baking sheet.
4. Bake in the oven for 18 minutes.

Buns with walnuts

Servings: 4

Cooking time: 40 minutes

Nutrients per one serving: Calories: 165 | Fats: 23.1 g | Carbs: 4.5 g | Proteins: 18 g

Ingredients:

- 5 eggs
- 3 tbsp almond flour
- 3 tbsp coconut flour
- 1 ½ tbsp psyllium
- 2 tbsp butter
- ½ cup yogurt
- ½ cup grated parmesan
- 2 tsp baking powder
- ½ cup walnuts
- ½ tbsp cumin (for decoration)

Cooking process:

1. The oven to be preheated to 190°C (375°F).
2. In a bowl, beat the eggs by a mixer until uniformity. Add soft butter, dry ingredients, yogurt, and crushed walnuts. Mix well. Add the grated parmesan. Leave the dough for 10 minutes.

3. Make the round buns with wet hands, and lay out them on the baking sheet covered with parchment.
4. Season with cumin and bake in the oven for 20 minutes.

Buns with poppy seeds

Servings: 1-2

Cooking time: 10 minutes

Nutrients per one serving: Calories: 89 | Fats: 13 g | Carbs: 3 g | Proteins: 7.1 g

Ingredients:

- 1 tbsp almond flour
- 1 tbsp coconut flour
    - 1 tsp butter
    - ½ tsp baking powder
    - 1 egg
    - 1 tbsp cream
    - ½ tsp poppy seeds
    - A pinch of salt

Cooking process:

1. Grease the silicone baking form.
2. Add the egg and cream. Mix everything until uniformity.
3. Pour the dough into a form and put in a microwave for 3 minutes.
4. Cut ready buns in half and fry in a dry frying pan for 1 minute.

Indian bread with greens

Servings: 6-8

Cooking time: 75 minutes

Nutrients per one serving: Calories: 94 | Fats: 17 g | Carbs: 4.6 g | Proteins: 4.5 g

Ingredients:

- ⅔ cup coconut flour
- 2 tbsp psyllium
- ½ cup coconut oil
- 2 ½ tbsp bran
- 1 ½ tsp baking powder
- 2 cups water
- ½ tsp salt
- A bunch of fresh cilantro
- ¼ cup butter

Cooking process:

1. Mix all dry ingredients, and add melted coconut oilin abowl. Boil water, add to the mass and knead the dough. Leave it for 5 minutes.
2. Divide the dough into 8 round pieces. Roll out each piece into a thin flat cake. Fry in a pan with coconut oil.
3. Put flat cakes on a plate. Melt the butter, and chop the cilantro. Lubricate bread by butter and sprinkle with greens.

DINNER

Expert: Microwave Bread

Serving Size: 4 small rounds

Nutritional Values: 2 g Net Carbs; 3.25 g Proteins; 13 g Fat;132 Calories

Ingredients:

- Almond flour - .33 cup
- Salt - .125 tsp
- Baking powder - .5 tsp
- Melted ghee – 2.5 tbsp.
- Whisked egg – 1
- Oil – spritz for the mug

Directions:

1. Grease a cup with the oil. Combine all of the fixings in a mixing dish and pour into the cup. Put the cup in the microwave. Set the timer using the high setting for 90 seconds.

2. Transfer the mug to a cooling space for 2-3 minutes. Gently remove from the bread and slice into 4 portions.

Paleo Bread – Keto Style

Servings: 1 loaf – 10 slices

Nutritional Values: 9.1 g Net Carbs ; 10.4 g Proteins; 58.7 g Fat; 579.6 Calories

Ingredients:

- Olive oil - .5 cup (+) 2 tbsp.
- Eggs – 3
- Almond milk/water - .25 cup
- Coconut flour - .5 cup
- Baking soda – 1 tsp.
- Almond flour – 3 cups
- Baking powder – 2 tsp.
- Salt - .25 tsp.
- Also Needed: Loaf pan – 9 x 5-inches

Directions:

1. Warm up the oven to 300°F. Lightly spritz the pan with olive oil.
2. Combine all of the dry fixings and mix with the wet to prepare the dough.
3. Pour into the greased pan and bake for 1 hour.
4. Cool and slice.

Sesame Seed Bread

Servings: 6

Nutritional Values: 1 g Net Carbs ;7 g Proteins; 13 g Fat; 100 Calories

Ingredients:

- Sesame seeds – 2 tbsp.
- Psyllium husk powder – 5 tbsp.
- Sea salt - .25 tsp.
- Apple cider vinegar – 2 tsp.
- Baking powder – 2 tsp.
- Almond flour – 1.25 cups
- Boiling water – 1 cup
- Egg whites – 3

Directions:

1. Heat up the oven to reach 350°F. Spritz a baking tin with some cooking oil spray. Put the water in a saucepan to boil.
2. Combine the psyllium powder, sesame seeds, sea salt, baking powder, and almond flour.
3. Stir in the boiled water, vinegar, and egg whites. Use a hand mixer (less than 1 min.) to combine. Place the bread on the prepared pan.
4. Serve and enjoy any time after baking for 1 hour.

THE KETO LUNCH

Creamy Avocado and Bacon with Goat Cheese Salad

Salad gets an upgrade when crave-able avocado and goat cheese are combined with crispy bacon and crunchy nuts. Fast and good for lunch or dinner.

Variation tip: use different fresh herbs in the dressing.

Prep Time: 10 minutes Cook Time: 20 minutes

Serves 4

What's in it

Salad:

- Goat cheese (1 8-ounce log)
- Bacon (.5 pound)
- Avocados (2 qty)
- Toasted walnuts or pecans (.5 cup)
- Arugula or baby spinach (4 ounces)

Dressing:

- One-half lemon, juiced
- Mayonnaise (.5 cup)
- Extra virgin olive oil (.5 cup)

- Heavy whipping cream (2 T)
- Kosher salt (to taste)
- Fresh ground pepper (to taste)

How it's made

1. Line a baking dish with parchment paper.
2. Preheat oven to 400 degrees F.
3. Slice goat cheese into half-inch rounds and put in baking dish. Place on an upper rack in preheated oven until

   golden brown.
4. Cook bacon until crisp. Chop into pieces
5. Slice avocado and place on greens. Top with bacon pieces and add goat cheese rounds.
6. Chop nuts and sprinkle on the salad.
7. For dressing, combine lemon juice, mayo, extra virgin olive oil and whipping cream. Blend with countertop or immersion blender.
8. Season to taste with kosher salt and fresh ground pepper.

Net carbs: 6 grams Fat: 123 grams

Protein: 27 grams

Sugars: 1 gram

KETO AT DINNER

Minute Steak with Mushrooms and Herb Butter

This dinner comes together fast. Perfect for busy weeknights.

Variation tip: try over any of your favorite vegetables.

Prep Time: 10 minutes Cook Time: 20 minutes Serves 4

What's in it

For steaks:

- Minute steaks (8 qty)
- Toothpicks (8 qty)
- Gruyere cheese, cut into sticks (3 ounces)
- Kosher salt (to taste)
- Fresh ground pepper (to taste)
- Butter (2 T)
- Leeks (2 qty)
- Mushrooms (15 ounces)
- Extra virgin olive oil (2 T)
- For herb butter:

- Butter (5 ounces)
- Minced garlic cloves (1 qty)
- Garlic powder (.5 T)
- Chopped parsley (4 T)
- Lemon juice (1 t)
- Kosher salt (.5 t)

How it's made

1. Combine all herb butter ingredients in a glass bowl. Set aside for at least 15 minutes.
2. Slice leeks and mushrooms. Sauté in extra virgin olive oil until lightly brown. Season with salt and pepper. Remove from skillet and keep warm.
3. Season steaks with salt and pepper. Place a stick of cheese in the center and roll up steaks, securing with a toothpick.
4. Sauté on medium heat for 10 to 15 minutes.
5. Pour pan juices on vegetables.
6. Plate steaks and vegetables and serve with herb butter.

Net carbs: 6 grams

Fat: 89 grams

Protein: 52 grams

Sugars: 2 grams

CPSIA information can be obtained
at www.ICGtesting.com
Printed in the USA
BVHW050801120521
607047BV00003B/413